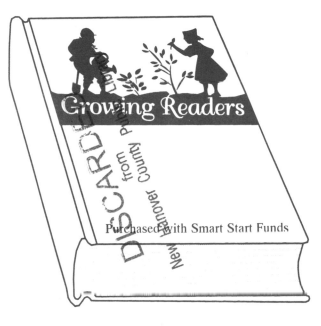

Growing Readers

Purchased with Smart Start Funds

NURSES

PEOPLE WHO CARE FOR OUR HEALTH

Robert James

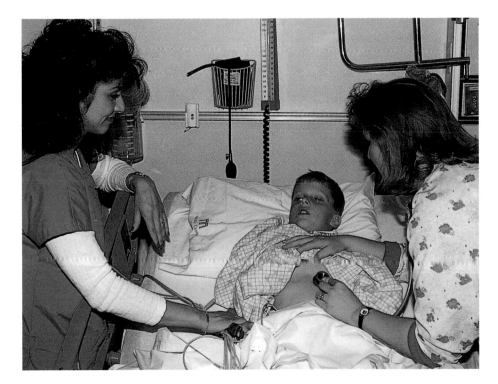

The Rourke Book Co., Inc.
Vero Beach, Florida 32964

PHOTO CREDITS
Cover, title page, pages 8, 12, 15, 17, 18, 21, © Kyle Carter;
page 4 © Hank Morgan/Rainbow; page 10 © Tom
McCarthy/Rainbow; pages 7, 13 courtesy Mercy Center, Aurora, IL

ACKNOWLEDGEMENTS
The author thanks Mercy Center, Aurora, IL, for its cooperation in
the publication of this book

Library of Congress Cataloging-in-Publication Data

James, Robert, 1942-
   Nurses / by Robert James.
      p. cm. — (People who care for our health)
   Includes index.
   Summary: Describes what nurses do, where they work, and how
they train and prepare for their jobs.
   ISBN 1-55916-167-1
   1. Nursing—Vocational guidance—Juvenile literature.
[1. Nursing—Vocational guidance. 2. Occupations.
3. Vocational guidance]
I. Title II. Series: James, Robert, 1942- People who care for our
health
RT61.5.J35 1995
610'.73'06'9—dc20   95–18940
                                         CIP
                                         AC

Printed in the USA

TABLE OF CONTENTS

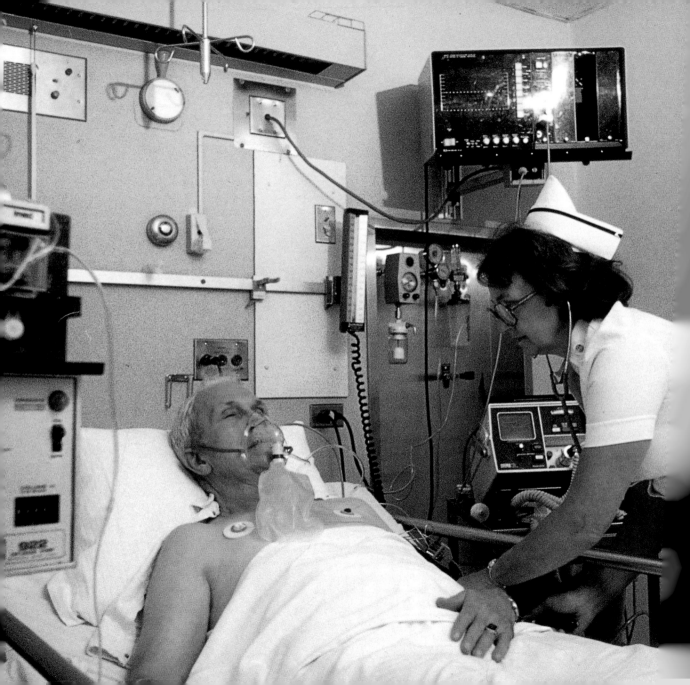

NURSES

Nurses today no longer wear only white. Nurses wear many different outfits. Nurses also perform many different jobs. One job that almost every nurse performs, though, is helping people who are ill or injured.

Nurses work as part of a team made up of health care **professionals** (pro FESH un ulz). These people are highly trained and skilled—doctors, nurses, **pharmacists** (FARM uh sists), **physical therapists** (FIZ uh kul THER uh pihsts), and others. These professionals work to help others regain and keep their health.

A nurse helps a patient in a hospital's intensive care unit

WHERE NURSES WORK

The main workplace of most nurses is a hospital. But nurses also work in dentist's offices, homes for elderly people, medical **clinics** (KLIN ihks), and schools. Nurses work in factories, mental hospitals, and on some ships and trains as well.

Nurses who work for government organizations may visit homes. Private nurses are hired by families to work in homes.

Nurses can watch the screens of machines that tell them how each patient's heart is performing in a hospita intensive care nursing station

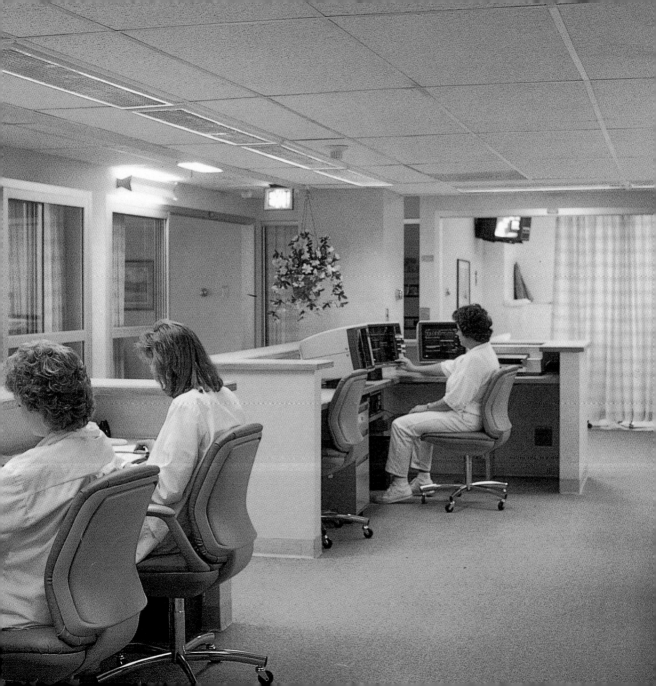

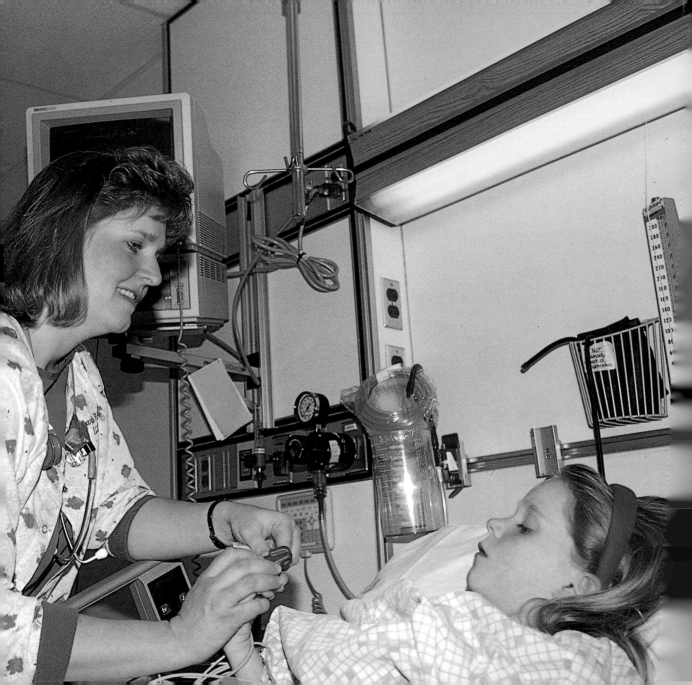

WHAT NURSES DO

Most nurses, of course, help take care of sick people. The exact kind of care a nurse provides depends upon the nurse's experience and education.

Nurses have many different levels of training. Some nurses are more highly trained than others.

Although most nurses work directly with patients, some nurses are teachers at schools of nursing. Others supervise, or watch over, the work of nurses.

Nurses deal with daily, even hour-to-hour care of patients

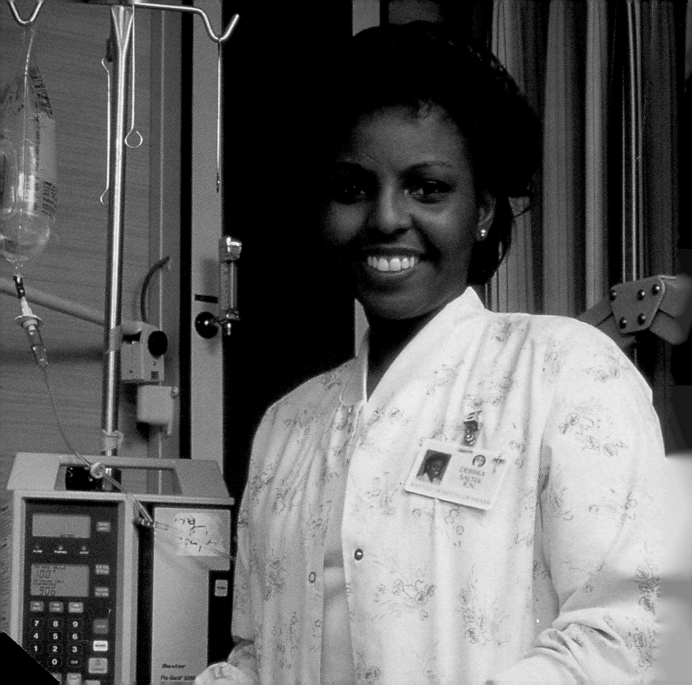

HOSPITAL NURSES

Hospital nurses work with patients in many different settings. Nurses are in a hospital's emergency (ER) and operating rooms (OR). They are in the hospital laboratories, exercise areas, and patient rooms.

Nurses are always "on call"—available when patients need them.

Nurses work closely with doctors. An operating room nurse, for example, must be able to follow a doctor's directions quickly and accurately.

11

Nurses' smiles give patients a daily lift

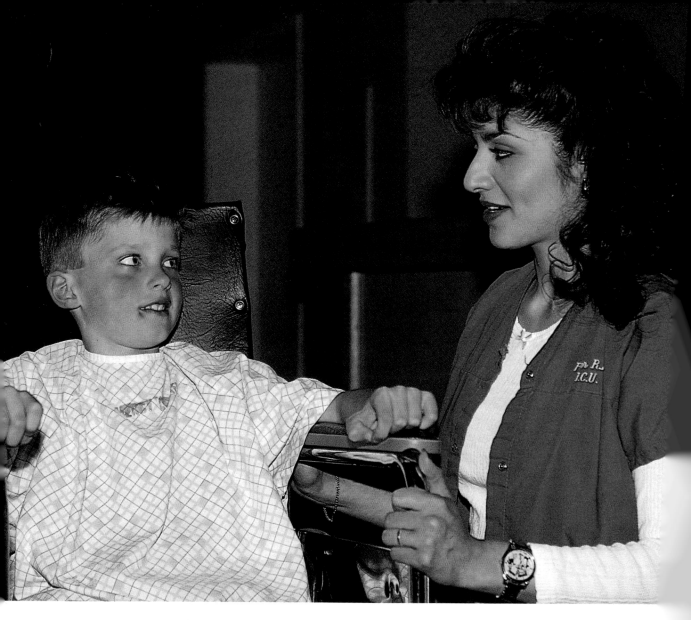

A nurse prepares her patient for a wheelchair ride

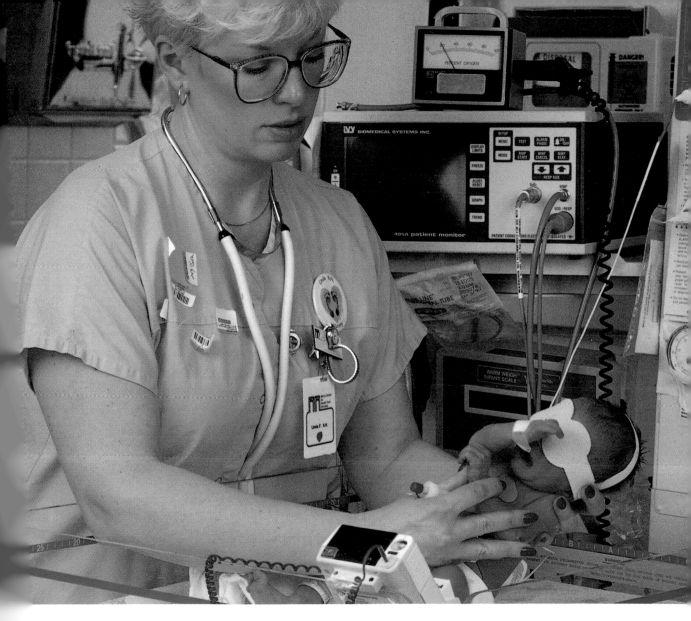

A hospital nursery nurse cares for an infant

NURSES AT WORK

Nurses help check the condition of patients. Nurses are always alert for signs of illness that may require a doctor's attention.

Nurses take a patient's blood pressure and **pulse** (PUHLSS). They draw blood samples, attach oxygen equipment, change dressings on wounds, and operate **intravenous** (in truh VEEN us), or IV, pumps.

Doctors determine what medicine a patient needs, but nurses give patients the medicine, often through needles.

A nurse checks her patient's blood pressure

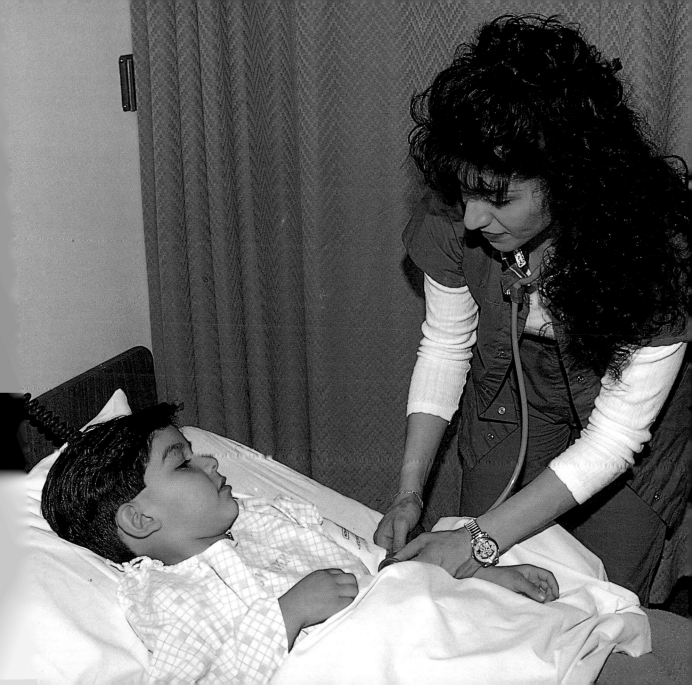

A FRIENDLY NURSE

Nurses know that a healthy mind helps make a healthy body. Nurses help their patients recover from physical problems. Cheery nurses, like good friends, also help people overcome feeling fearful, nervous, and low. Nurses help mend minds as well as bodies.

Nurses counsel patients about their illnesses. They help many patients feel better about themselves. Nurses also encourage patients to make changes in their lifestyles so that they will keep their health.

A patient listens to her own heartbeat with the nurse's stethoscope

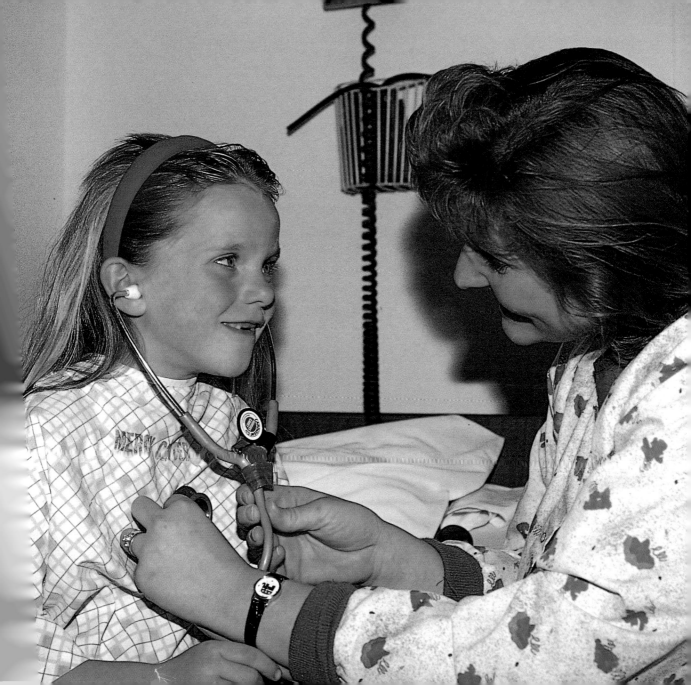

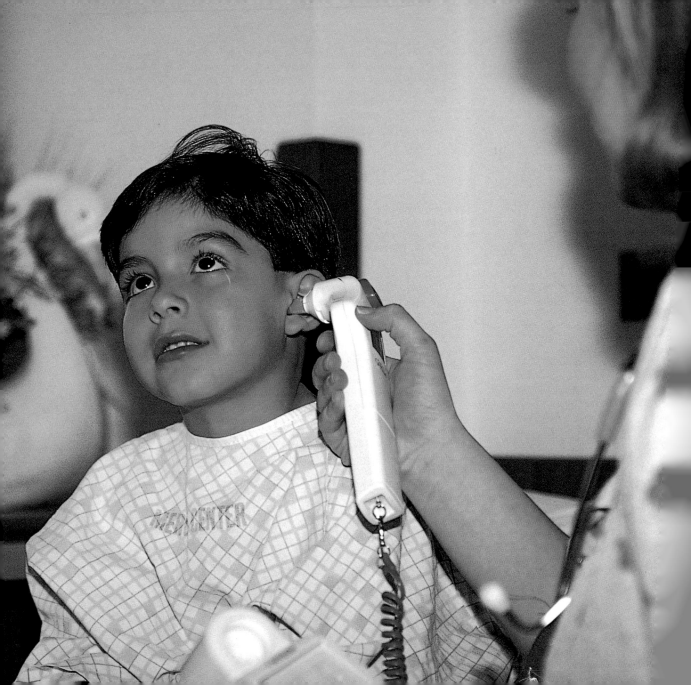

A NURSE'S TOOLS

Nurses are trained to work with many medical instruments and machines. Nurses often use blood pressure cuffs, stethoscopes, needles, and thermometers.

Nurses in special parts of a hospital, such as the Intensive Care Unit (ICU), work with special instruments. ICU nurses assist people who have very serious illnesses. The nurses work with such instruments as **respirators** (RES per a terz) and EKG monitors. The EKG monitor measures a patient's heart activity.

A nurse checks the patient's temperature

A NURSE'S HELPERS

Nurses assist doctors and other health care professionals. Nurse's aides help nurses.

Aides take over jobs that require little training, such as making a patient's bed, bathing a patient, and feeding a patient. With help from an aide, a nurse can spend more time on the tasks that require greater skill.

Young **volunteer** (vol un TEER) workers, called "candy stripers," because of their bright uniforms, help hospital nurses, too.

Working together as health-care team members, a nurse (left) and docto discuss a patient's health record

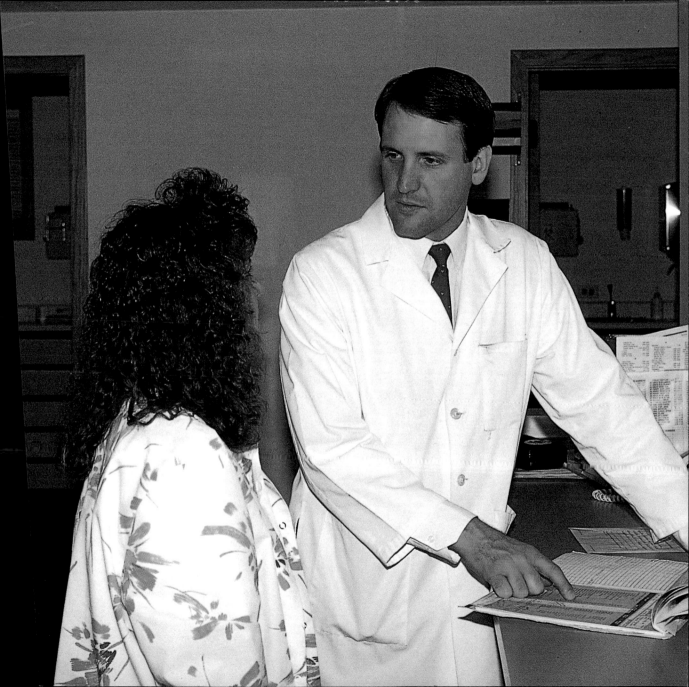

BECOMING A NURSE

A professional, or registered, nurse (RN), must graduate from a nursing program in college or special nursing school. Programs last two to five years.

Nurse practitioners are professional nurses who take certain advanced studies beyond those of RN's.

Licensed practical nurses (LPN's) graduate from a 12-month nursing program.

Since Florence Nightingale began the first school of nursing in 1860, nursing has been largely a "woman's job." Today, however, about one nursing student in 15 is a man.

Glossary

clinic (KLIN ihk) — a place, usually with several doctors, for treating large numbers of patients who don't need overnight care

intravenous (in truh VEEN us) — anything that works through the body's veins, such as a liquid pumped through an intravenous (IV) tube

pharmacist (FARM uh sist) — one who studies and prepares drugs

physical therapist (FIZ uh kul THER uh pihst) — a health care professional who practices physical therapy, a type of treatment

professional (pro FESH un ul) — one who is highly trained, highly skilled, and paid for his or her work

pulse (PUHLSS) — the up-and-down movement in the wrist and elsewhere caused by the heartbeat

respirator (RES per a ter) — a machine used to help people breathe

volunteer (vol un TEER) — one who without pay willingly performs a task that he of she offers to do

INDEX